TOP 13 SUPERFOODS THAT WILL BOOST YOUR METABOLISM

THE ROLE OF SUPERFOODS IN WEIGHT MANAGEMENT

DOROTHY ROBERTS MEREDITH

TABLE OF CONTENTS

INTRODUCTION

Welcome to the Top 13 Superfoods to the Top 13 Superfoods That Will Boost Your Metabolism. My name is Dorothy Roberts Meredith and I'm excited to share this book with you. We all know that eating more fruits and vegetables is good for your health. The right fuel in your body makes you feel vibrant on every level. You feel stronger, more empowered, you even get healthier looking skin. I started a plan that changed my life, and this has been my journey.

In a world where health and wellness are more important than ever, understanding how to optimize your body's natural process is key to achieving your goals. Metabolism, the complex set of chemical reactions that connect food into energy, plays a crucial role in our overall health, weight management, and vitality.

If you find yourself feeling sluggish and unmotivated, despite your best efforts to eat healthy and you continue to struggle with low energy levels, cravings for unhealthy snacks, and a slower metabolism that seem to be holding you back from reaching your Fitness goals, it is time to make a change. I decided to delve deeper into the world of nutrition and explore superfoods that could boost my metabolism.

After researching various options, I made a commitment to incorporate these top 13 superfoods into my daily meals. Each week, I focus on one or two superfoods, including green tea, chili peppers, grapefruits and experimenting with creative recipes and snacks that feature these nutrient powerhouses. Within just a few weeks, I started to notice significant changes. Drinking a cup of green tea in the morning replaced my usual coffee ritual and gave me a clean energy boost without the jitters. Adding Chili Peppers to my meals not only spiced things up but also curb my appetite, making me feel full for a longer period of time. I Incorporated grapefruit into my breakfast routine, enjoying it alongside yogurt and granola, which became one of my favorite ways to start the day.

Ultimately, this experience taught me the importance of fueling my body with the right foods. By embracing these 13 super foods, I successfully revamped my diet, boosted my metabolism, and improved my overall well-being. My journey with superfoods not only transformed my physical health but also inspired me to share my story with others, hoping to encourage them to try these powerful foods as well.

In this book, you will discover 13 incredible superfoods that not only taste delicious but also work wonders for your metabolism. These nutrient-dense foods are packed with vitamins, minerals, and antioxidants that can help enhance your metabolic rate, promote fat burning, and support overall energy levels.

Whether you're looking to shed a few pounds, gain energy, or simply incorporate healthier choices into your diet, this guide will provide you with valuable insights and practical tips. It's not that hard to substitute metabolism boosting foods for those that aren't so healthy and to add a few calorie smart items to your meals. Choosing calorie burning foods instead of the ones that just turn to Fat will make a huge difference in your weight loss program. You can change the way you look at food by adding more fruits and vegetables into your daily meal planning.

There are many ways to eat superfoods in one serving. You may be able to maximize your consumption of superfoods by combining them. So nourish to flourish by incorporating the power of superfoods for Optimum Health. Ways to incorporate different superfoods into one meal include preparing:

- Bowl
- Smoothie
- Soup
- Salads

Each super food offers distinct nutritional benefits, but in general they are known to:

- Reduce inflammation in the body
- Boost heart health
- Promote a strong immune system
- Lower cholesterol
- Lessen the risk of cancer

When combined in the diet, these ingredients can create a synergistic effect, enhancing your metabolic rate and potentially aiding in weight management. However, it's important to remember that while these foods can support metabolism, they work best as part of an overall balanced diet and healthy lifestyle, including regular physical exercise.

Incorporating these Superfoods into your diet can provide numerous health benefits and enhance overall well-being. The recipes included not only incorporate your specified ingredients but also balance flavors. These recipes are not only delicious but also packed with nutrients from these amazing superfoods! enjoy!

It is with great pleasure that I share with you these 13 superfoods that will boost your energy and increase your metabolism thereby helping you lose unwanted weight. Each chapter highlights a specific superfood detailing its unique benefits.

Join me on this journey to unlock the power of these superfoods and transform your approach to nutrition and embracing the delicious possibilities ahead, let's Kickstart your metabolism together!

Here's to your health and happiness!

Dorothy Roberts Meredith

1

GREEN TEA

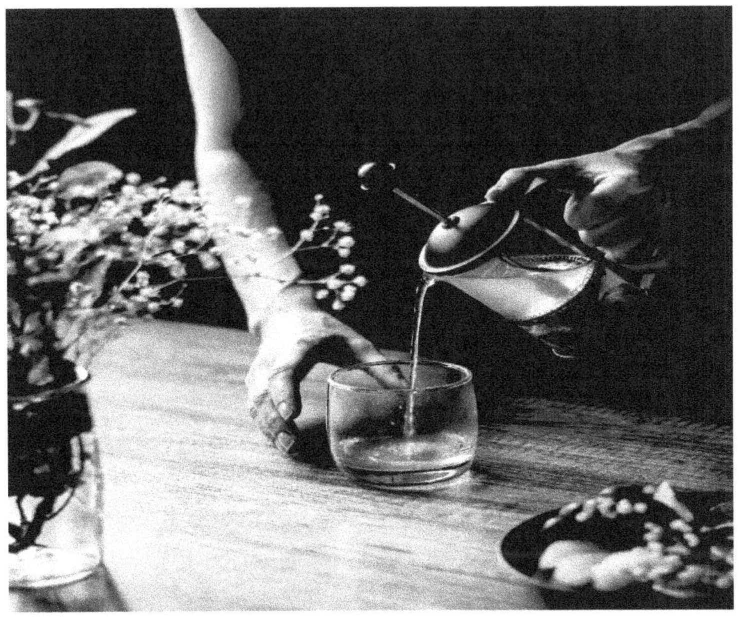

Like hot peppers, green tea speeds up your heart rate, leading to a higher metabolism. Not only does the caffeine in green tea kickstart your heart, it also frees up stores of fatty acids so they can be burned as fuel. The secret ingredient and green tea is the compound ECGC, which not only spikes metabolism, it tells the brain and nervous system to work faster. Green tea is a great substitute for calorie fielded soft drinks or lattes since it's loaded with antioxidants. Rich in antioxidants and catechins, green tea can enhance metabolic rate and promote fat oxidation.

HEALTH BENEFITS:

1. **Rich in Antioxidants:** Contains polyphenol, particularly cations, which help reduce oxidative stress and inflammation in the body.
2. **Supports Heart Health:** Regular consumption may lower cholesterol levels and improve cardiovascular health.
3. **Improves brain function:** Contains L-Theanine, which, in accommodation with caffeine, can enhance cognitive function and mood.
4. **May aid in weight management:** Green tea can help with fat loss, especially during exercise.

Matcha Green Tea also provides a more sustained and steady energy release without the crash that often accompanies coffee. The combination of caffeine and L-Theanine in Matcha can really help you feel alert and focused throughout the day.

HOW IT BOOSTS YOUR METABOLISM:

- **Catechins in green tea:** Can enhance fat oxidation and increase metabolic rate. Green tea is rich in catechins, particularly epigallocatechin gallate (EGCG), Which can increase energy expenditure and fat oxidation. Studies have shown that the consumption of green tea can boost metabolic rate for a short period of tim
- **Caffeine:** Green tea contains caffeine, which may enhance fat burning and improve exercise performance, further supporting weight management.

INCORPORATING IT INTO YOUR DIET:

- **Iced tea:** Brew a batch of iced tea for a refreshing drink. You can add slices of lemon, mint, or fruits for extra flavor.
- **Soups and broths:** Add brewed tea to soups or broths as a flavorful liquid base.
- **Tea infused desserts:** Incorporate tea into desserts like tea flavored ice cream, cake, or cookies for a unique twist.

Green Tea Smoothie:

Ingredients:

- 1 cup brewed green tea (Cooled)
- 1 banana

- ½ cup spinach
- ½ cup frozen berries (blueberries or strawberries)
- 1 tablespoon honey (optional)
- Ice cubes

Instructions:

1. Brew green tea and let it cool
2. in a blender, combine all ingredients and plan until smooth
3. adjust sweetness with honey if desired. serve chilled

CHILI PEPPERS

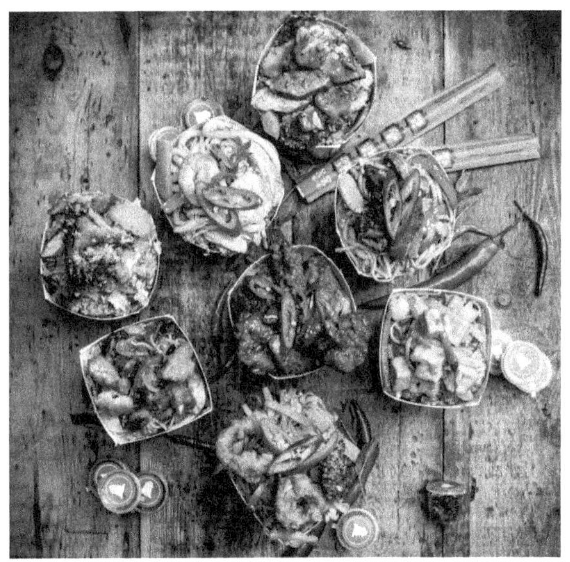

Although they aren't high in protein, hot peppers like jalapeños, habaneros and Thai Chilies can kick up your metabolism by speeding up your heart rate. Consuming a very spicy meal can boost your metabolism by up to 25% for as long as three hours, so it's a good idea to always have some Sriracha or Tabasco sauce, handy to heat up dishes that need a little spice. Peppers can be part of an Asian stir-fry or add zing to homemade chili. Containing capsaicin, Chili Peppers can increase calorie burn and promote a filling of fullness, which may Aid weight management. No food can be bland or boring. If you turn up the temperature with high peppers!

HEALTH BENEFITS:

1. **Contains Capsaicin:** This compound gives chili peppers their heat and is known to boost metabolism by increasing energy expenditure.
2. **Pain Relief:** Capsaicin has analgesic properties and may help reduce pain when used topically.
3. **Anti-Inflammatory:** Chili peppers can help lower inflammation in the body.
4. **Promotes Digestive Health:** May stimulate digestive enzymes and promote a healthy gut.
5. **Boosts Immunity:** High vitamins A and C, which support immune function.

HOW IT BOOSTS YOUR METABOLISM:

- **Capsaicin:** The active compound in chili peppers, capsaicin, has thermogenic properties, meaning it can increase body temperature and boost calorie burning. It may also help reduce appetite, leading to lower overall calorie intake.

- **Metabolic boost:** Capsaicin can stimulate the production of adrenaline, which enhances metabolic rate temporarily.

INCORPORATING IT INTO YOUR DIET:

- **Cooking with chili peppers:** Add fresh or dried chili peppers to stir-fries, stews, or sauces for heat and flavor.
- **Spicy marinades:** Create marinades for meats or tofu that include chili paste or chopped Chili Peppers to add spiciness.
- **Salsa and Dips:** Make homemade salsa or guacamole with diced Chili Peppers for a spicy kick.
- **Chili oil:** Drizzle chili oil on pizza, pasta, or roasted vegetables to enhance flavor.
- **Stuffed peppers:** Stuffed bell peppers with a mixture of grains, beans, and spices, and add chopped Chili Peppers for it and extra spice level.

Spicy chili pepper and ginger stir-fry

Ingredients:

- 1 tablespoon olive oil
- 1 bell pepper, sliced
- 1 zucchini, sliced
- 1 cup broccoli florets
- ½ fresh chilies peppers, sliced (Adjust based on spice preference)

- 1 tablespoon fresh ginger, minced
- 2 tablespoons soy sauce or Tamari
- Cooked brown rice or quinoa for serving

Instructions:

1. Heat olive oil in a pan over medium Heat
2. Add bell pepper, zucchini, and broccoli; stir fry for about 5 minutes
3. Add the sliced Chili Peppers and minced ginger; cook for another 2-3 minutes
4. Stir in soy sauce and serve over brown rice or quinoa

GRAPEFRUIT

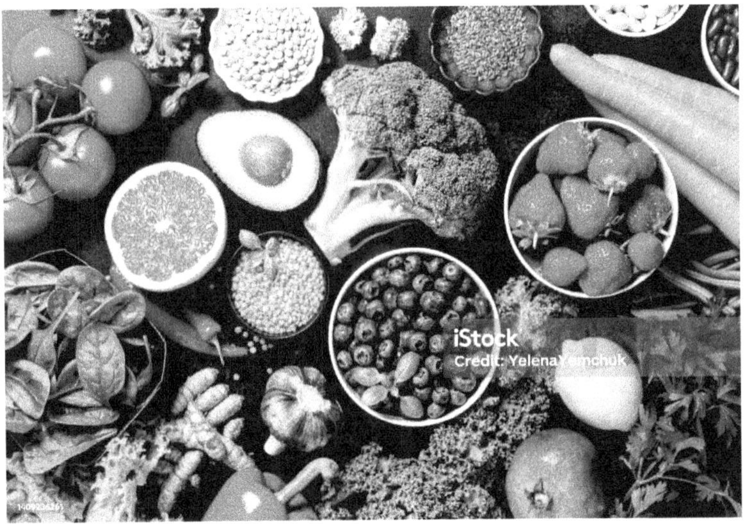

Although it's bitter taste can be a bit much at times, research shows that adding citrus to your menu may boost your immune system, support weight loss and even keep you regular. Rio Red grapefruits are sweeter and much more tolerable. However, grapefruits can interfere with some medications like cholesterol and diabetes drugs, so be sure to consult a healthcare provider to learn more about interactions. Grapefruits are high in fiber, so it slows down the absorption of sugars into the bloodstream, which helps to curve blood sugar spikes. This fruit can help regulate insulin levels and has been linked to weight loss, making it beneficial for metabolism.

HEALTH BENEFITS:

1. **Rich in Vitamins and Nutrients:** High in vitamin C, vitamin A and antioxidants that support overall health.
2. **Weight Management:** Studies suggest that consuming grapefruit can lead to weight loss, possibly due to its impact on insulin levels
3. **Heart Health:** May lower cholesterol levels in blood pressure, reducing the risk of heart disease.
4. **Boost Immune System:** High water content helps keep you hydrated.
5. **Supports Digestive Health:** Rich in fiber, grapefruit can promote healthy digestion.

HOW IT BOOSTS YOUR METABOLISM:

- **Naringin:** Grapefruit contains naringin, A flavonoid that may help regulate insulin levels and improve the metabolism. Balancing insulin levels can prevent fat storage and promote weight loss.
- **Fiber:** The fiber content in grapefruit can help improve digestion and promote a feeling of fullness, potentially leading to reduced calorie intake.

INCORPORATING IT INTO YOUR DIET:

- **Smoothies:** Playing grapefruit segments with other fruits, yogurt, and spinach or kale for a refreshing smoothie.
- **Avocado toast:** Top avocado toast with sliced grapefruit for a tangy twist.
- **Grain bowls:** Add grapefruit to grain bowls with quinoa, black beans, avocado, and a light dressing.
- **Fruit platter:** Include grapefruit slices on a fruit platter with other fresh fruits for a refreshing snack option.
- **Citrus fish:** Top grilled or baked fish with grapefruit salsa or segments for a vibrant dish.

Grapefruit and Berry Salad:

Ingredients:

- 1 grapefruit, segmented
- 1 cup mixed berries {strawberries, blueberries, raspberries)
- 1 tablespoon honey or maple syrup
- 1 fresh mint leaves for garnish
- (Optional): feta cheese or goat cheese for added flavor

Instructions:

1. In a bowl, combine grapefruit segments and mixed berries
2. Drizzle with honey or maple syrup and toss gently
3. Garnish with fresh mint leaves and cheese if using, serve immediately or chilled
4. Toss gently to combine without breaking the berries

BERRIES: (STRAWBERRIES, BLUEBERRIES, RASPBERRIES, ACAI BERRIES)

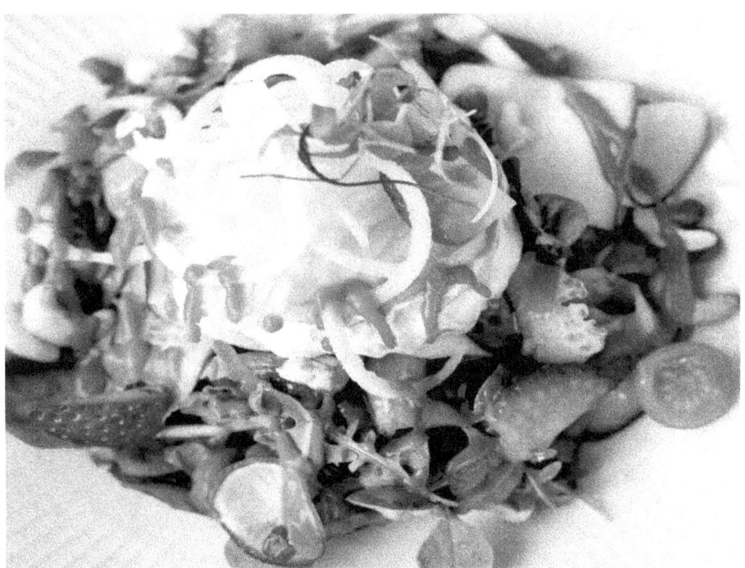

Different types of berries have different qualities and amounts of nutrients. For example, raspberries are low in sugar and contain antioxidant levels, while blueberries contain more sugar than other berries. Berries provide potassium, magnesium, vitamins C and K, fiber, probiotics and carbohydrates that help promote a healthy gut. Recent studies show that blueberries in particular, May reduce the risk of breast cancer, improve cardiovascular health and slow down. Cognitive decline in the elderly. It is known that a Acia Berry contains omega-9, a fatty acid and powerful anti-inflammatory, and has antioxidant levels, higher than cranberries, raspberries, blackberries, strawberries, or blueberries. Low in calories and high in fiber, berries like blueberries, Acai berries, and strawberries are nutrient dense and support metabolic health. Because of their high antioxidant levels, these berries also support heart and brain health.

HEALTH BENEFITS:

1. **High in Antioxidants:** Packed with vitamins, minerals, and antioxidants that combat oxidative stress.
2. **Support heart health:** Can improve cholesterol levels and lower blood pressure.
3. **Anti-inflammatory properties:** Helps reduce inflammation, which is linked to various chronic diseases.
4. **Supports cognitive function:** May enhance brain health and memory due to their antioxidant properties.
5. **Digestive health:** High in fiber, good at helping to maintain healthy digestion.

HOW IT BOOSTS YOUR METABOLISM:

- **Antioxidants:** Berries are high in antioxidants such as anthocyanins, which may help improve metabolic health and reduce inflammation. Reducing inflammation can lead to better metabolic function.
- **Fiber:** Like grapefruit, berries are also high in fiber, which can help slow digestion and promote satiety, aiding and weight management.

INCORPORATING IT INTO YOUR DIET:

- **Smoothies:** Blend a mix of Berries (Strawberries, Blueberries, Raspberries, Blackberries) with yogurt, milk, or a dairy-free alternative for a nutritious smoothie.
- **Oatmeal:** Top your morning oatmeal with fresh or frozen berries for added flavor and nutrients.
- **Pancakes or Waffles:** Add berries to pancake or waffle batter, or just use them as a topping with a drizzle of maple syrup.
- **Frozen berries:** Keep frozen berries on hand for a quick snack. they're great on their own or blended into smoothies.
- **Sauces and Glaze:** Use berries to make sauces or glazes for meats like chicken or pork.

Berry Chia Pudding:

Ingredients:

- 1 cup almond milk (or any milk of choice)
- ¼ cup chia seeds
- 1 tbsp sweetener (honey, maple syrup, or agave)
- 1 cup mixed berries
- Optional toppings: nuts, coconut flakes

Instructions:

1. In a bowl, whisk together almond milk, Chia seeds, and sweetener
2. Cover and refrigerate for at least 4 hours or overnight until it thickens
3. Before serving, top with mixed berries and additional toppings if desired

GINGER

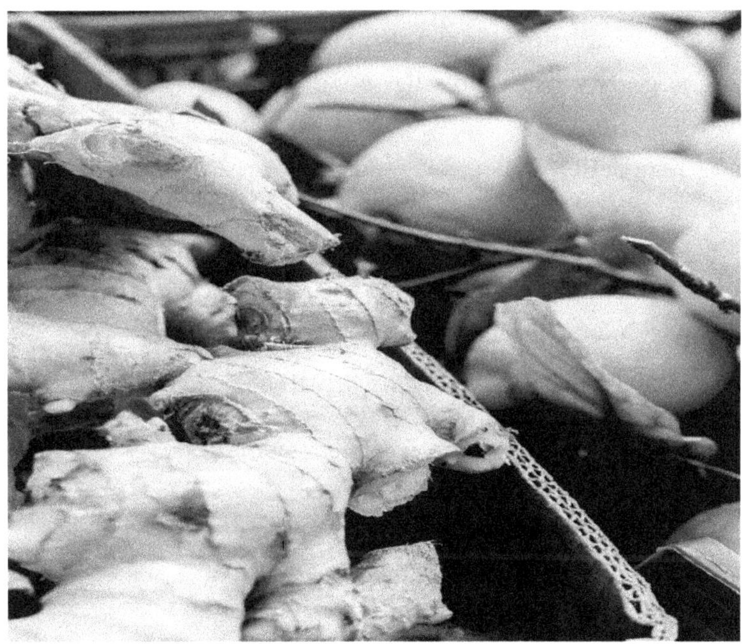

There are certain chemical compounds in fresh ginger that help your body ward off germs. They are good at halting growth of bacteria, and they may also keep viruses like RSV at bay. Ginger's anti-inflammatory agents help reduce swelling. This may be especially helpful for treating symptoms of both Rheumatoid arthritis and Osteoarthritis. Ginger's antibacterial power can also keep your mouth healthy. Active compounds called gingerol keep oral bacteria that can cause periodontal disease, a serious gum infection, from growing. Known for its digestive benefits, gender can also enhance metabolic rate and help burn more calories after meals.

HEALTH BENEFITS:

1. **Anti-inflammatory:** Contains gingerol, which has powerful anti-inflammatory effects.
2. **Digestive Aid:** helps alleviate nausea, bloating, and digestion.
3. **Pain relief:** May reduce muscle pain and soreness after exercise.
4. **Supports immune system:** Antioxidant properties can help fight infections and boost immunity.
5. **May lower blood sugar levels:** Some studies suggest ginger can improve insulin sensitivity and lower blood sugar levels.

HOW IT BOOSTS YOUR METABOLISM:

- **Thermogenic effect:** Ginger can have a thermogenic effect similar to chili peppers, potentially increasing calories expenditure and fat burning.

- **Digestive Aid:** Ginger has been shown to improve digestion and nutrient absorption, supporting overall metabolic processes.

INCORPORATING IT INTO YOUR DIET:

- **Stir-fries:** Add fresh or minced ginger to stir fries for a spicy kick and flavor.
- **Soups:** Incorporate Ginger into soups, especially Asian inspired ones like miso soup or Thai coconut soup.
- **Marinades:** Use ginger in marinades for meat and tofu. It pairs well with soy sauce, garlic, and citrus.
- **Curries:** Add Ginger to Curries for depth and warmth. it works great in both Indian and Thai Foods
- **Baking:** Incorporate ground ginger into baked goods such as cookies, cakes, or muffins for a warm spiciness.
- **Salad dressings:** Whisk grated Ginger into vinaigrettes for salads.

Ginger Tea with Honey and Lemon

Ingredients:

- 1 inch piece of fresh ginger, sliced
- 2 cups water
- Juice of 1 lemon
- Honey to taste

Instructions:

1. Boil water and add Ginger slices, let it simmer for about 15 minutes
2. Stir the tea into a cup and add lemon juice and honey to taste
3. Serve warm as a soothing drink

Ginger-Infused green tea with chili:

Ingredients:

- 2 cups of water
- 2 green tea bags
- 1 tablespoon fresh ginger, sliced
- 1/2 fresh chili peppers, sliced (Adjust based on spice preference)
- Honey or agave syrup to taste (Optional)

Instructions:

1. Boil the water in a pot
2. Add Ginger and chili peppers, and let it simmer for about 5 minutes
3. Remove from heat and add the green tea bags; steep for 3 to 5 minutes
4. Remove tea bags and strain the mixture to remove Ginger and chili slices
5. Sweetened with honey or agave syrup if desired. serve hot or iced with lemon slices

6

GREEK YOGURT

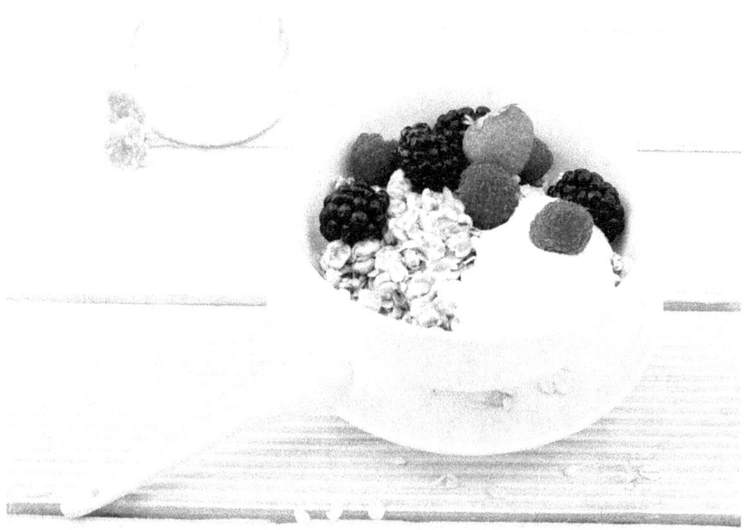

Besides being thick and creamy, this tasty Dairy tree packs a whopping 18 g of protein in a 6 oz serving. serve it with your favorite fruit or substitute for sour cream and recipes for dips. Because Greek yogurt is high in protein and probiotics, it can boost metabolism by promoting muscle growth and improving gut health.

HEALTH BENEFIT:

1. **High protein content:** Provides a good amount of protein, which can help with muscle repair and satiety.
2. **Probiotics:** Contains live cultures that promote good health and may improve digestion.
3. **Calcium:** A good source of calcium, important for bone health.
4. **Low in sugar:** Compared to flavored varieties of yogurt, plain greek yogurt has less sugar, especially the unsweetened varieties.

HOW IT BOOSTS YOUR METABOLISM:

- **High in protein:** Greek yogurt is an excellent source of protein, which helps build and repair tissues and can increase feelings of fullness.
- **Probiotics:** It contains live cultures that can benefit gut health by promoting a healthy balance of bacteria in the digestive system.
- **Calcium and nutrients colon:** Greek yogurt is rich in calcium, which is essential for bone health, as well as vitamins like B12 and phosphorus.

INCORPORATING IT INTO YOUR DIET:

- **Smoothie Bowl:** Blend Greek yogurt with your favorite fruits and top with granola, nuts, and seeds.

- **Veggie dip:** Combine Greek yogurt with herbs and spices (like dill or garlic) for a healthy dip for veggies.
- **Pancakes:** Substitute Greek yogurt for some of the liquid in your pancake batter for extra protein and a fluffy texture.
- **Salad dressing:** Use Greek yogurt as a base for creamy dressings instead of mayonnaise or sour cream.
- **Marinades:** Use Greek yogurt as a base for a marinating meat: it helps tenderize and add flavor.

Greek yogurt parfait

Ingredients:

- 1 cup Greek yogurt (Plain or flavored)
- 1/2 cup granola (your choice)
- 1/2 cup mixed berries (strawberries, blueberries, raspberries, etc.)
- 1 tablespoon honey or maple syrup (optional)
- A Sprinkle of nuts or seeds (optional)
- Mint leaves (for garnish, (optional)

Instructions:

1. In a bowl, add half of the Greek yogurt as the first layer.
2. Add granola, sprinkle half of the granola on top of the yogurt layer.
3. Add berries and layer half of the mixed berries over the granola.

4. Repeat layers, repeat the layers with the remaining Greek yogurt, granola, in berries.
5. Drizzle with sweetener (optional) Drizzle honey or maple syrup on top.
6. Add nuts / seeds (optional) Layer half of the mixed berries over the granola.
7. Garnish (optional), add a few mint leaves for a refreshing touch.
8. Serve immediately, enjoy your delicious Greek yogurt parfait immediately, or refrigerate for a short time until ready to eat.

EGGS

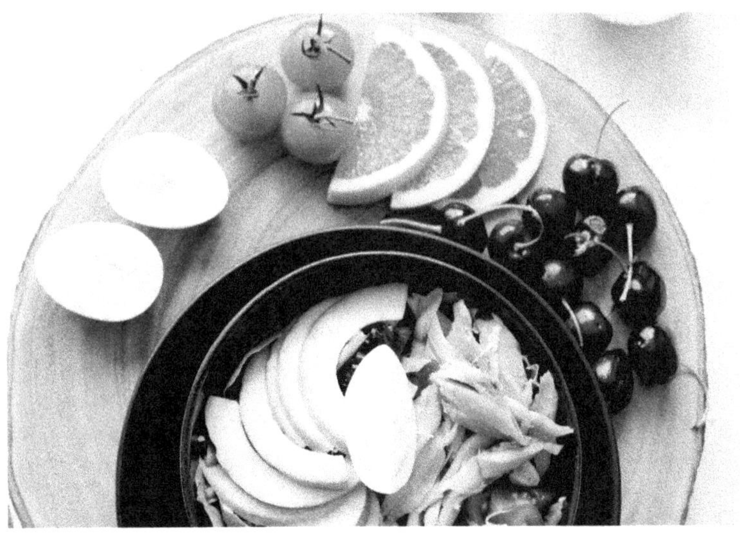

The egg is one of Nature's most perfect foods, with two packing 12 G of protein. Four egg whites have 14 G of protein, so it's a great substitute for meat. add veggies and low-fat cheese for a tasty omelet, or chop-boiled eggs with mustard, spices and yogurt for a Tangy egg salad. Eggs are a great source of high-quality protein; eggs can support muscle maintenance and promote a higher metabolic rate. spinach

HEALTH BENEFIT:

1. **Nutrient-Dense:** Eggs containing Central nutrients, including vitamins D and B12, selenium, and choline, important for brain health.
2. **High-Quality Protein:** They provide high quality protein that contains all essential amino acids.
3. **Healthy fat:** Rich in monounsaturated and polyunsaturated fats, beneficial for heart health. Eggs have healthy fats, including omega-3 fatty acids, especially if you choose eggs from pasture raised hens

HOW IT BOOSTS YOUR METABOLISM:

- **Complete protein** Eggs are considered a complete protein source, providing all nine essential amino acids needed by the body.
- **Rich in nutrients:** They contain important nutrients like vitamin d, B vitamin (especially B12), selenium and choline, which support brain health.

INCORPORATING IT INTO YOUR DIET:

- **Omelets:** Fill an omelet with your favorite ingredients such as spinach, mushrooms, cheese, or ham.

- **Egg muffins:** Mix beaten eggs with vegetables, cheese, and meats, pour into muffin tins, and bake.
- **Eggs benedict:** Make a healthier version with whole grain English muffins, poach eggs, and a light hollandaise or avocado sauce.
- **Frittatas:** Bake a frittata with eggs, vegetables, and cheese for a filling lunch option.
- **Quiche:** Make a crustless quiche with eggs, cream, veggies, and cheese for a delicious dinner dish.

Egg and Greek yogurt breakfast bowl:

Ingredients:

- 1 cup cooked quinoa or brown rice
- 1 soft boiled egg
- ½ cup Greek yogurt
- Add your choice of veggies (spinach, or cherry tomatoes and avocado)

Instructions:

1. In a bowl, layer the quinoa or rice, Greek yogurt, chopped veggies, and sliced avocado.
2. Top with the soft-boiled egg and season with salt, pepper, and a drizzle of olive oil.

Veggie packed egg muffins:

Ingredients:

- 6 large eggs
- ½ cup milk (Or dairy-free alternative)

- 1 cup spinach
- ½ Bell pepper, diced (any color)
- ½ cup cherry tomatoes, halved
- 1/4 cup onion, diced
- ½ cup shredded cheese (cheddar, feta, or your choice)
- Salt and pepper to taste
- Olive oil or cooking spray (for grease in the muffin pan)

Instructions:

1. Preheat oven to 350 Fahrenheit
2. Grease a muffin tin with olive oil or cooking spray
3. In a large mixing bowl, whisk together the eggs and milk. Season with salt and pepper
4. Stir in chopped spinach, Bell pepper, cherry tomatoes, onion, and shredded cheese until well combined.
5. Pour the egg mixture evenly into the muffin cups, feeling each about 2/3 full.
6. Bake in the preheated oven for 18-20 minutes, or until the muffins are set and slightly golden on top.
7. Allow muffins to cool for a few minutes before gently removing them from the pan.
8. Serve: Enjoy warm or store it in an airtight container in the refrigerator for up to a week. You can reheat them in the microwave when ready to eat.

SPINACH

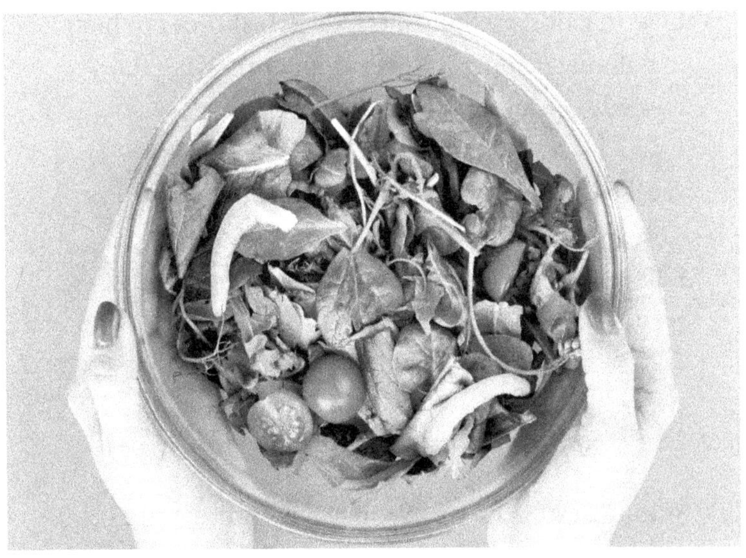

This leafy green is a powerhouse, packing 5 grams of protein into one cup of cooked spinach. mixed with mushrooms and vinaigrette for a nutrient packed salad or steamed with garlic. spinach is also a great addition to lentil and other soups. It can be consumed raw or cooked.

HEALTH BENEFIT:

1. **Rich in Vitamins and Minerals:** A great source of vitamin A, C, K, and minerals like iron and magnesium.
2. **Antioxidants:** Contains antioxidants such as lutein and zeaxanthin that are beneficial for eye health.
3. **Low in calories:** Low-calorie food that can promote weight management.

HOW IT BOOSTS YOUR METABOLISM:

- **Low in calories:** Spinach is low in calories but high in volume, making it a great food for feeling full without consuming too many calories.
- **Packed with vitamins and minerals:** It's an excellent source of vitamins A, C, and K, as well as iron and magnesium.
- **Fiber:** Fiber and spinach is digestion and can help regulate blood sugar levels.

INCORPORATING IT INTO YOUR DIET:

- **Smoothies:** Blend fresh spinach with fruits like banana, mango, or berries, along with yogurt or almond milk for a nutritious smoothie.
- **Breakfast bowls:** Create a bowl with quinoa or brown rice topped with sauteed spinach, poached eggs and avocado.

- **Soups:** Stir fresh or frozen spinach into soups or stews just before serving for added nutrition.
- **Salads:** Use fresh spinach as a base for salads. top it with nuts, seeds, cheese, fruits, and your favorite dressings.
- **Casseroles:** Incorporate spinach into casseroles or lasagna for a hidden veggie boost.

Spinach and feta egg muffins:

Ingredients:

- Six large eggs
- 1 cup fresh spinach, chopped
- ½ cup feta cheese, crumbled
- Salt and pepper to taste

Instructions:

1. Preheat the oven to 350 Fahrenheit and grease a muffin pan.
2. In a bowl, whisk together the eggs, then mix in the spinach, feta, salt, and pepper.
3. Pour the egg mixture into the muffin tin, filling each cup about 3/4 full.
4. Bake for 20-25 minutes until the eggs are set. let cool slightly before removing from the pan.

9

LEAN PROTEIN

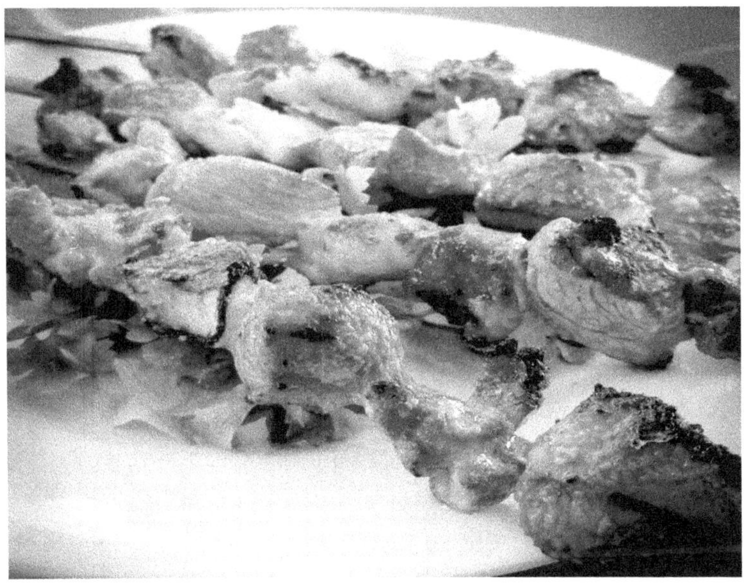

Don't think you have to ban all Meats from your weight loss program. Lean cuts of beef or poultry can kick up your metabolism because the body burns up energy digesting lean protein. Plus eating lean protein can help to build and preserve muscle mass, and that's what burns the calories and fat. Look for skinless chicken breasts and the least fatty curves of beef.

HEALTH BENEFIT:

1. **Muscle maintenance:** Essential for building and maintaining muscle mass.
2. **Weight Management:** Can promote a feeling of fullness, aiding and weight control.
3. **Variety of sources:** Includes poetry, legumes, tofu, and low-fat dairy, offering diapers options for meals.

HOW IT BOOSTS YOUR METABOLISM:

- **Thermic effect of food:** Digestion requires energy, and protein has a higher thermic effect compared to fats and carbohydrates, this means that your body uses more energy to digest, absorb, and process proteins, which can increase your metabolic rate temporarily after you eat.
- **Muscle mass maintenance:** Consuming lean proteins supports Muscle maintenance and growth. Muscle tissue is metabolically active, meaning it burns more calories at rest compared to fat tissue. An increase in muscle mass can lead to a higher resting metabolic rate.
- **Satiety and appetite control:** Lean proteins can promote feelings of fullness and reduce hunger, which may help control overall calorie intake. When you feel satiated, you're less likely to overeat or snack

on high calorie foods, contributing to better weight management and metabolism regulation.

- **Blood sugar regulation:** Lean proteins can help stabilize blood sugar levels by slowing down the digestion and absorption of carbohydrates. This can prevent spikes and crashes in blood sugar, which may help regulate hunger and energy levels, ultimately supporting a healthy metabolism.
- **Hormonal balance:** Protein consumption can influence hormones related to hunger and metabolism, such as insulin and glucagon. Proper hormonal balance is essential for Effective metabolism and energy utilization.

Incorporating it into your Diet:

- **Grilled chicken:** Marinate and grilled chicken breast serving it with quinoa and steamed vegetables.
- **Stir fry:** Use lean cuts of beef or turkey in a stir fry with mixed vegetables and a light sauce.
- **Bean chili:** Prepare a vegetarian chili using beans for a filling and protein-rich option.

Grilled lemon herb chicken breast:

Ingredients:

- 4 boneless, skinless chicken breasts
- 3 tbsp olive oil
- Juice of two lemons
- 4 cloves garlic, minced
- 1 teaspoon dried oregano

- 1 teaspoon dried thyme
- Salt and pepper to taste
- Fresh parsley for garnish

Instructions:

1. **Marinate chicken:** In a bowl, mix Olive oil, lemon juice, garlic, oregano, thyme, salt, and pepper. Add chicken breast and marinate for at least 30 minutes (Or up to overnight in the fridge).
2. **Preheat grill:** Preheat your grill or grill pan over medium-high heat.
3. **Grilled chicken:** Remove chicken from marinade, shaking off excess. grilled chicken for 6 to 7 minutes on each side or until fully cooked (internal temperature should reach 165° F/75C).
4. **Serve:** Let rest for a few minutes, then slice and garnish with fresh parsley. Serve with a side of steamed vegetables or salad.

10

LEAN FISH / SALMON

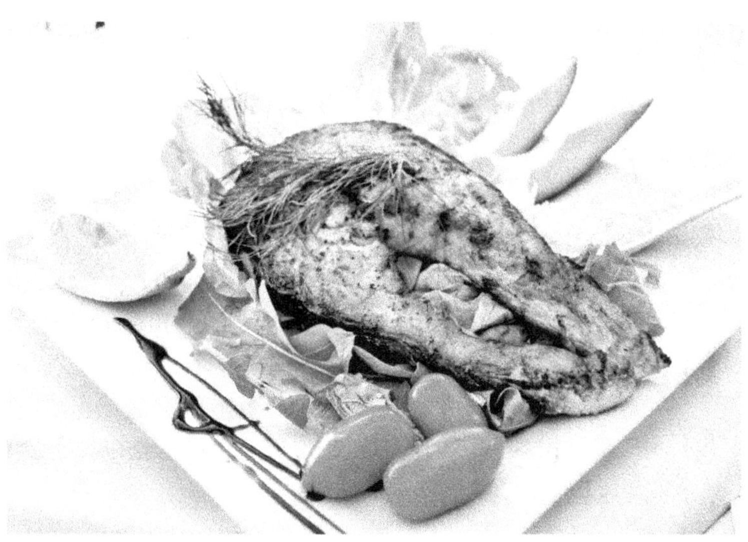

With 28 grams of protein per 6 oz, Seafood is a great catch. Cold water fish varieties like salmon, tuna, trout and mackerel are rich inl omega-3 fatty acids and have been shown to boost your metabolism by as much as 400 calories a day. Try 3 to 5 servings per week, and prepare your Seafood in a healthy manner, like grilling or broiling rather than frying. Tuna salad made with low fat Mayo is a healthier choice for sandwiches than fatty lunch and meats.

HEALTH BENEFIT:

1. **Heart Health, Omega-3 fatty acids:** Rich and omega-3 fatty acids, which are beneficial for heart health and brain function.
2. **High quality protein:** Provides a good source of protein, essential for overall bodily functions like muscle growth and repair.
3. **Rich in Vitamins and minerals:** Fish is packed with essential vitamins and minerals, including vitamin d, B12, selenium, and iodine, which support various bodily functions, from bone health to immune function.
4. **Support brain function:** The Omega-3 fatty acids found in fish are crucial for brain health and cognitive function. They have been linked to reduced risk of cognitive decline and they also help improve mood.
5. **Weight management:** Lean proteins, including fish, can help with weight management by promoting fullness and reducing overall calorie intake.

TYPES OF LEAN FISH:

- **White fish:** Card, haddock, and tilapia are examples of lean white fish that are low in calories and fat.
- **Fatty fish:** Salmon, trout, and sardines, while higher

in fat, provide beneficial omega-3 fatty acids and are still considered healthy options.

- **Shellfish:** Shrimp, crab, and scallops are also lean protein sources that can be included in a balanced diet.

HOW IT BOOSTS YOUR METABOLISM:

- **High in protein:** Salmon and other fish are high-quality proteins, which has a thermogenic effect. This means that your body burns more calories digesting protein compared to fats or carbohydrates. Your body expends more energy to digest them. Salmon is rich in omega-3 fatty acids, which have been shown to improve metabolic Health by reducing inflammation, increasing insulin sensitivity, and promoting fat loss. Omega-3s may also enhance the metabolic Effect of exercise.
- **Omega-3 fatty acids:** The healthy fats in fish and salmon help reduce inflammation and may promote metabolic health. Omega-3s are also linked to improve insulin sensitivity, which can assist in maintaining a healthy weight.

INCORPORATING IT INTO YOUR DIET:

- **Baked salmon:** Season and bake salmon, serving it with roasted vegetables and brown rice or quinoa.
- **Salmon salad:** Use quinoa as a base for salads, mixing with vegetables and a protein source.

- **Fish tacos:** Use screwed or baked salmon and tacos with cabbage slaw and avocado.
- **Shrimp tacos:** Season shrimp with taco seasoning and use cabbage slaw and avocado on corn or flour shell.

Lemon garlic butter baked cod:

Ingredients:

- 4 cod filets
- 3 tbsp butter, melted
- 3 cloves garlic, minced
- Juice of one lemon
- Salt and pepper, to taste
- fresh parsley, chopped (for garnish)

Instructions:

1. **Preheat oven:** Preheat your oven to 400 degrees Fahrenheit
2. **Prepare baking dish:** Grease a baking dish with cooking spray or a little Olive oil.
3. **Make the sauce:** In a bowl, mix melted butter, garlic, lemon juice, salt, and pepper.
4. **Arrange fish:** Place the cod filets in the prepared baking dish and pour the lemon garlic sauce over them
5. **Bake:** Bake for 12-15 minutes, or until the fish is cooked thoroughly and flakes easily with a fork.
6. **Garnish:** Sprinkle with fresh parsley before serving.

11

QUINOA

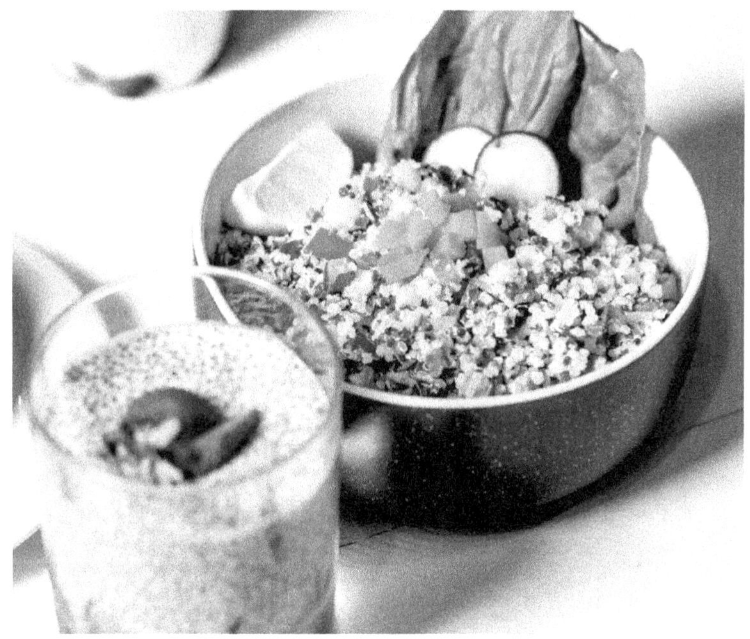

Quinoa is a high protein whole grain that takes more energy to digest, quinoa can help increase metabolic rate and keep you satisfied longer and is gluten-free. Incorporating quinoa into your Diet can not only enhance flavor and variety but also provide an array of health benefits that contribute to overall well-being.

HEALTH BENEFIT:

1. **High in fiber:** Quinoa is rich in dietary fiber, which age digestion, helps maintain bowel health, and can assist in weight management by promoting a feeling of fullness.

2. **Rich in nutrients:** Quinoa is packed with vitamins and minerals, including magnesium, iron, potassium, phosphorus, zinc, and B vitamins. These nutrients play various roles in bodily functions, including energy production, immune function, and Bone health.

3. **Antioxidant properties:** Quinoa contains antioxidants such as quercetin and kaempferol, which help reduce oxidative stress and inflammation in the body, potentially lowering the risk of chronic disease.

4. **Gluten free:** Quinoa is naturally gluten-free, making it an excellent option for those with celiac disease or gluten sensitivity.

5. **Bone health:** Granola is a good source of magnesium and phosphorus, both of which are important for maintaining strong bones.

6. **Heart health:** The fiber, antioxidants, and healthy fats found in quinoa may contribute to improved heart health by reducing cholesterol levels and lowering blood pressure.

HOW IT BOOSTS YOUR METABOLISM:

- **Complete protein:** Quinoa is a complete protein, containing all nine essential amino acids. Consuming adequate protein can increase the thermic effect of food (TEF), leading to increased calorie burning after meals.
- **Complex carbohydrates:** Quinoa is a whole grain that provides complex carbohydrates and fiber, helping to stabilize blood sugar levels and provide sustainable energy without causing spikes and hunger.

INCORPORATING IT INTO YOUR DIET:

- **Salads:** Use cooked quinoa as a base for salads, adding vegetables, beans, nuts, and dressing of your choice for a nutritious meal.
- **Soups and Stews: Add** Quinoa to soups and stews for extra texture and nutrients. it works well as a thickener as well.
- **Breakfast bowls:** Cook quinoa and almond milk or other plant-based milks and topped with fruits, nuts and seeds for a healthy breakfast option.
- **Quinoa burgers:** Mix cooked corn with beans, vegetables, and spices to create delicious vegetarian burgers.
- **Side dishes:** Serve quinoa as a side dish, seasoned with herbs and spices, instead of rice or pasta.
- **Stir-fries:** At quinoa to stir-fried vegetables and proteins for a healthy and colorful meal.

- **Baking:** East granola flower in baking recipes to increase the nutrient content of Breads and baked goods.

Seasoned Quinoa

Ingredients:

- 1 cup quinoa
- 2 cups water or vegetable broth
- 1/4 teaspoon salt and pepper (optional)

Instructions:

1. **Rinse the quinoa:** Place the quinoa in a fine mesh strainer and rinse it under cold running water for about 2 minutes. This helps remove any bitterness.
2. **Cook the canola:** in a medium saucepan, combine the rinsed quinoa, water (or broth), and salt, bring to a boil over medium-high heat. Once it reaches a boil, reduce the heat to low, cover, and let it simmer for about 15 minutes, or until all the liquid is absorbed
3. **Fluff and served:** Remove the saucepan from heat and let it sit for 5 minutes with the lid on. Fluff the corner with a fork before serving.

KALE

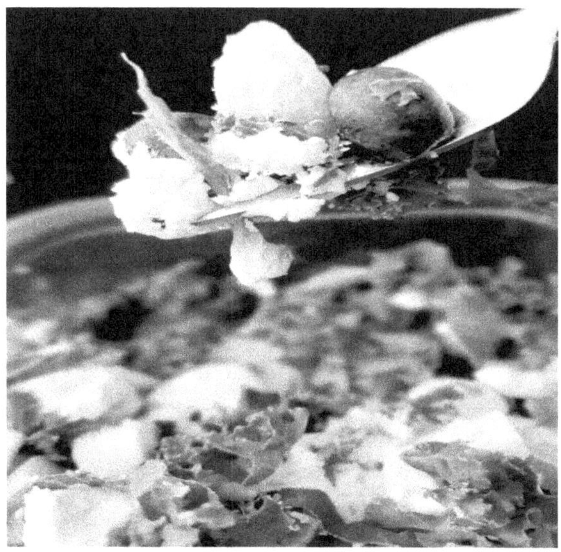

K ale is a nutrient-dense leafy green vegetable that offers numerous Health benefits. Incorporating kale into your diet can be easy, whether in salads, smoothies, soups, or as a cook side dish. just remember to wash it thoroughly before consuming.

HEALTH BENEFIT:

1. **Rich in nutrients:** Carol is a Powerhouse of vitamins and minerals, including vitamins A, C, and K, as well as calcium, potassium and magnesium.
2. **High in antioxidants:** Kale is loaded with antioxidants like quercetin and kaempferol, which help combat oxidative stress and inflammation in the body.
3. **Supports heart health:** The fiber, potassium, and antioxidants and kale can contribute to improved heart health by reducing cholesterol levels, lowering blood pressure, and supporting overall cardiovascular function
4. **Anti-inflammatory properties:** The various compounds found in kale, including omega-3 fatty acids and vitamins, can help reduce inflammation in the body.
5. **Bone health:** Kale is an excellent source of vitamin K, which is essential for bone health and helps with calcium abortions, potentially reducing the risk of fractures.
6. **Weight management:** Being low in calories but high in fiber in water content, kale can help you feel full and satisfied, making it a great addition to a weight loss diet

HOW IT BOOSTS YOUR METABOLISM:

- **High nutrient density:** Kale is low in calories but high in vitamins, minerals, and antioxidants. This nutrient density means that you can consume it without significantly increasing your calorie intake, while still providing your body with the nutrients it needs to function optimally.

- **Rich in fiber:** Kale is a good source of dietary fiber, which is digestion and helps regulate blood sugar levels. A high fiber diet can support a healthy metabolism by improving gut health and promoting a sense of fullness, which may reduce overall calorie consumption.
- **Supports muscle health:** Kate contains important nutrients like protein, iron, and various vitamins that support muscle function and recovery. Having some muscle mass can lead to a higher resting metabolic rate, meaning you'll burn more calories even when at rest.
- **Antioxidants and anti-inflammatory properties:** Kale is rich in antioxidants, which can help reduce inflammation in the body. Chronic inflammation can negatively impact metabolism and contribute to weight gain. By reducing inflammation, kale may help improve metabolic functions.
- **Thermogenic effect:** Foods that are harder to digest, like those rich in fiber and nutrients, can cause your body to expand more energy during digestion. This thermogenic effect can provide a slight boost to your metabolic rate.
- **Hydration:** Kale has a high-water content, which can contribute to overall hydration. Staying well hydrated is essential for maintaining an efficient metabolism, as dehydration can slow down metabolic processes.

- **Low glycemic index:** Kale is a low glycemic index, meaning it doesn't cause rapid spikes and blood sugar levels. Stable blood sugar levels can help maintain energy levels and prevent cravings, supporting better metabolic health.

INCORPORATING IT INTO YOUR DIET:

- **Kale Chips:** Make your own kale chips by tossing kale leaves into Olive oil, seasoning, and baking them until crispy. This makes for a healthy snack!
- **Soups and stews:** And chopped kale to soups and stews. It works well in vegetable, being, or chicken soups, providing extra vitamins and texture.
- **Omelets and Scrambled:** Mix kale into omelet or scrambled eggs. sauté the kale first, then add it to your eggs for a nutritious breakfast.
- **Casseroles:** Incorporate kale into casseroles or baked dishes. It can add flavor and nutrition to recipes like lasagna or quinoa bake.

Garlic sauteed kale:

Ingredients:

- 1 bunch of kale (about 6-8 cups chopped)
- 2 Tablespoons olive oil
- 3 cloves garlic, minced
- ½ tsp red pepper flakes (optional for heat)
- Salt and pepper to taste
- Lemon wedges (for serving)

Instructions:

1. **Prepare the kale:** Wash the kale thoroughly under cold water to remove any dirt or regret. remove the tough stems and chop the leaves into bite-sized pieces.
2. **Heat the oil:** In a large Skillet or sauté pan, heat the oil over medium heat.
3. **Sauté the garlic:** Add the minced garlic to the pan and sauté for about 1-2 minutes until fragrant, being careful not to let it burn.
4. **Add kale:** Add the chopped kale to the pan, if the skillet is crowded, you can add it in batches. stir well to coat the kale and the oil and garlic.
5. **Cook the kale:** Sauté the kale for about 5-7 minutes, stirring occasionally, until it's wilted and tender.
6. **Season:** Season with salt, peppers, and red pepper flakes (if using) to taste. give it a final stir.
7. **Serve:** Remove from heat and serve warm, garnish with lemon wedges. squeeze fresh lemon juice over the top for added flavor!

AVOCADO

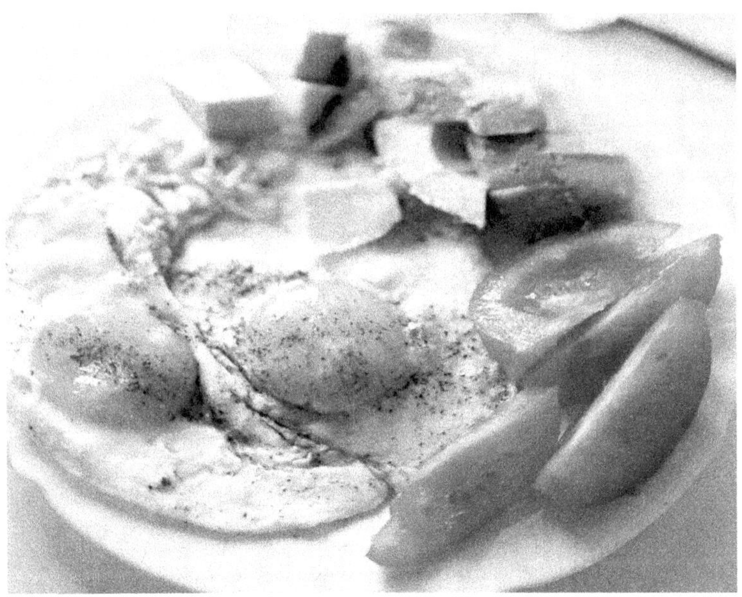

This delicious creamy green fruit is packed with nutrients including two grams of protein per half, and those two grams contain all 9 essential amino acids as well as omega-3 fatty acids that are great for your heart. Avocado has a healthy fat and is fiber rich. Avocados contain Prebiotics, which support the growth of beneficial gut bacteria, contributing to overall gut health. It has numerous health benefits.

HEALTH BENEFIT:

1. **Rich in nutrients:** Avocados are packed with vitamins and minerals, including vitamin K, vitamin E, vitamin C, B vitamins (especially B6 and folic), and potassium.
2. **Heart health:** Avocados are high in monounsaturated fats, particularly oleic acid, which can help reduce bad cholesterol levels (LDL) and lower the risk of heart disease.
3. **High in fiber:** Avocados are a great source of dietary fiber, which AIDS digestion, promotes regular bowel movements, and help maintain a healthy weight by keeping you for longer.
4. **Antioxidant properties:** They contain antioxidants such as lutein and zeaxanthin, which are beneficial for Eye Health and may help reduce the risk of age-related macular Degeneration.
5. **Anti-inflammatory effects:** The healthy fats, vitamins, and phytochemicals in avocados have anti-inflammatory properties that may help reduce inflammation in the body.
6. **Healthy skin and hair:** The vitamins and healthy fats in avocados contribute to healthy skin and hair, and they are often used in beauty products for moisturizing effects.

HOW IT BOOSTS YOUR METABOLISM:

- **Healthy fats:** Avocados are rich in mono on saturated fats, which can help increase energy expenditure, healthy fats can also provide a longer lasting source of energy compared to refined carbohydrates.
- **High fiber content:** the fiber in avocados AIDS digestion and promotes feelings of fullness, which can help regulate appetite and prevent overeating. A balanced appetite can lead to better weight management, indirectly supporting metabolic health.
- **Stable blood sugar levels:** The combination of healthy fats and fiber can stabilize blood sugar levels, preventing spikes and crashes that can affect energy levels and metabolism.
- **Hormonal balance:** Healthy fats from avocados can support hormone production, including hormones involved in metabolism and fat storage.

INCORPORATING IT INTO YOUR DIET:

- **Salads:** Add diced or sliced avocados to salads for a creamy texture and added nutrients
- **Toast:** Spread mashed avocado on whole grain toast. You can top it with toppings like sliced tomatoes. radishes. poached eggs. Or a sprinkle of chili flakes.
- **Smoothies:** Blend avocado into your smoothies for a creamy consistency and a boost of healthy fats. It goes well with fruits like bananas, spinach, and berries.

- **Sushi:** Include avocado and sushi rolls for added creaminess.
- **Sandwiches and wraps:** Use avocado slices as a condiment and sandwiches and wraps instead of mayonnaise or butter.
- **Dips and spreads:** Blend avocado with yogurt or cream cheese to create a rich dip or spread for crackers and veggies.

Guacamole:

Ingredients:

- 2 ripe avocados
- 1 small onion, finely chopped
- 1-2 cloves of garlic, minced
- 1 medium tomato, DIC
- Juice of one line adjust to taste
- Salt, to taste
- Fresh cilantro, chopped optional
- Jalapeno, finely chopped optional for spice

Instructions:

1. **Prepare the avocados:** Cut the avocado in half, remove the pit, and scoop the flesh into a mixing bowl.
2. **Mash the avocados:** Use a fork or a potato masher to mash the avocados to your desired consistency (smooth or chunky).

1. **Add ingredients:** Start in the finely chopped onion, minced garlic, diced tomato, lime juice, and salt. If you like heat, add some finely chopped jalapeno.
2. **Mix well:** Combine everything until well mixed. taste and adjust seasoning, adding more lime or salt if needed.
3. **Garnish:** If using cilantro, fold it and gently.
4. **Serve:** Enjoy your guacamole with tortilla chips, on tacos, or as a topping for your favorite dishes.

PLEASE LEAVE A REVIEW

If you found this book helpful, I would greatly appreciate it if you could leave a positive review on Amazon by simply scanning the QR Code. Thank you in advance.

Click here to leave a review

CONCLUSION

In conclusion, the journey through the vibrant world of superfoods reveals not just an array of colors and flavors, but also a transformative approach to Health and Wellness each superfood, whether it's the antioxidant rich berries, the nutrient dense kale, or the protein packed quinoa, contributes uniquely to our wellbeing. The warming spice of Chili Peppers invigorates our metabolism, while the soothing properties of Ginger aid digestion, reminding us that food is not only sustenance but also medicine. Incorporating lean proteins, eggs, and fish into our diet provides essential building blocks for our bodies, supporting both strength and vitality. Meanwhile, the creamy richness of Greek yogurt and the healthy fats from avocados nourish and satisfy our cravings in the most wholesome way. Spinach and green tea invite us to embrace the greens, offering a treasure trove of vitamins and antioxidants that can enhance our energy and focus.

As we continue to explore the profound impact of these superfoods on our lives, it becomes clear that embracing a holistic approach to nutrition can revolutionize our overall well-being. Each bite offers the potential for vitality, supporting not just our physical health, but also our mental clarity and emotional resilience. Imagine starting each day with the breakfast bowl adorned with creamy Greek yogurt, topped with vibrant berries, a sprinkle of quinoa, and a perfectly poached egg. This simple yet nutritious meal embodies the essence of superfood synergy, fueling our body with the essential nutrients required to thrive. As we cultivate our awareness of food choices, we begin to see cooking as a creative outlet not just a necessity. Infusing our meals with spices like ginger and chili peppers not only enhances flavor but also amplifies Health benefits, turning ordinary dishes into powerful allies for our wellness journey.

Furthermore, integrating these superfoods into our daily routines encourages us to reconnect with nature. Choosing fresh whole ingredients like leafy greens, citrus fruits, and wholesome proteins fosters a sense of gratitude for the earth's bounty and the nourishment it provides. This connection is vital in today's fast-paced world, reminding us to slow down and savor the experience of eating mindfully.

In conclusion, the 13th superfoods we've explored lay the groundwork for a healthier lifestyle that honors both our bodies and the environment. By prioritizing these nutrient-dense foods, we unlock the potential for greater energy, improved mood, and enhanced longevity. Let this book serve not only as a guide to delicious, heartful eating but also as an invitation to embark on a continuous journey towards wellness, a journey that begins with every delicious bite we take.

As we cultivate habits that include these superfoods, we Empower ourselves to take charge of our health, embracing a lifestyle that celebrates balance, nourishment, and vitality. By making conscious choices and exploring the Myriad ways these ingredients can be integrated into our meals, we embark on a lifelong journey of wellness, ready to face life challenges with energy and resilience. So let us raise our Bowl filled with the goodness of superfoods together, let's celebrate the power of superfoods and commit to nourishing ourselves in a way that brings us joy, vitality and a deeper connection to the world around us, here's to a life filled with flavor, health, and happiness one superfood at a time!

RESOURCES

Asana Rebel - Get in shape. (n.d.). https://asanarebel.com/

Prevention.com - health advice, nutrition tips, trusted medical information. (n.d.-b). Prevention. https://prevention.com/

WebMD - Better information. Better health. (2024, September 10). WebMD. https://webmd.com/

Know more. Feel better. (n.d.). Verywell Health. https://verywellhealth.com/

Health News - Medical News today. (n.d.). https://medicalnewstoday.com/

Welcome to good food. (n.d.-b). Good Food. https://www.bbcgoodfood.com/

Healthline: Medical information and health advice you can trust. (n.d.). Healthline. https://healthline.com/